21-DAYS FULL-BODY DETOX DIET

Transform your body in 21-days: discover a full-body detox diet for renewed energy, weight loss and vibrant health with easy-to-follow recipes

Odesa Mulan

Table of Contents

CHAPTER ONE 5

Introduction to Full Body Detox: Understanding Its Importance

....5

The Concept of Full Body Detox 5

Understanding Toxins and Their Impact 6

Importance of Full Body Detox...6

Conclusion 8

CHAPTER TWO 9

Preparing for Your Detox Journey: Mental and Physical

Readiness 9

Cultivating a Positive Mindset..10

Embracing Self-Care Practices 11

Addressing Underlying Health Issues 11

Preparing Your Environment...12

Conclusion 12

CHAPTER THREE 13

Meet Your Detox Guide: Dr. Barbara's Background and

Expertise...13

Dr. Barbara's Educational Background 13

Professional Experience and Clinical Practice 14

Areas of Expertise..15

Conclusion 16

CHAPTER FOUR 17

The Science Behind Detoxification: How It Benefits Your Body
....17

Understanding Detoxification Pathways 18

Liver Detoxification...18

Key Players in Detoxification..18

Benefits of Detoxification 19

Conclusion 21

CHAPTER FIVE 22

Day 1-7: Cleansing Phase - Removing Toxins from Your System
....22

Understanding the Cleansing Phase 22

Strategies for Optimal Detoxification............................23

Conclusion 25

CHAPTER SIX 26

Day 8-14: Rejuvenation Phase - Replenishing Nutrients and
Energy 26

Key Objectives of the Rejuvenation Phase 27

Strategies for Rejuvenation..27

Conclusion 29

CHAPTER SEVEN 30

Day 15-21: Transformation Phase - Integrating Healthy Habits for Long-Term Wellness 30

Key Objectives of the Transformation Phase 31

Strategies for Transformation 31

CHAPTER EIGHT...34

Essential Foods for Detox: Exploring Nutrient-Rich I€ngredients 34

Conclusion 37

CHAPTER NINE 38

CHAPTER TEN 42

Maintaining Your Results: Tips for Sustaining a Healthy Lifestyle After the Detox 42

BONUS: SOME HERBAL AND HOLISTIC APPROACHES TO KNOW 45

THE END...82

COPYRIGHT © 2023

CHAPTER ONE

Introduction to Full Body Detox: Understanding Its Importance

Detoxification, a process aimed at eliminating toxins from the body, has gained significant traction in recent years as individuals become increasingly conscious of their health and well-being. Among the various forms of detoxification, full body detox stands out as a comprehensive approach targeting the entire organism. In this discourse, we delve into the intricacies of full body detox, elucidating its importance and the mechanisms underlying its efficacy.

The Concept of Full Body Detox

Full body detoxification revolves around the principle of purging accumulated toxins from all bodily systems, including the liver, kidneys, colon, skin, and lymphatic system. Unlike localized detox methods that target specific organs or functions, such as liver detox or colon cleansing, a full body detox aims for holistic purification. It recognizes the interconnectedness of bodily systems and seeks to restore equilibrium by addressing toxic overload comprehensively.

Understanding Toxins and Their Impact

Toxins are substances that exert harmful effects on the body, often disrupting physiological processes and predisposing individuals to various ailments. They can originate from external sources such as environmental pollutants, pesticides, heavy metals, and food additives, as well as internal factors like metabolic byproducts and stress-induced chemicals. Prolonged exposure to toxins can overwhelm the body's natural detoxification pathways, leading to toxin accumulation and subsequent health issues.

The accumulation of toxins in the body can manifest in diverse ways, ranging from fatigue, digestive disturbances, and skin disorders to more severe conditions like autoimmune diseases, hormonal imbalances, and cancer. Moreover, toxins can impair cellular function, compromise immune responses, and contribute to chronic inflammation, which underlies many degenerative diseases. Therefore, mitigating toxin burden through full body detox holds immense therapeutic potential in promoting overall health and vitality.

Importance of Full Body Detox

1. **Enhanced Vitality and Energy:** By alleviating the burden of toxins, a full body detox rejuvenates cellular function and metabolic processes, leading to increased energy levels and vitality. As the body becomes free from toxic overload, individuals often experience improved stamina, mental clarity, and overall well-being.

2. **Optimized Organ Function:** Full body detox supports the optimal functioning of vital organs involved in detoxification, such as the liver, kidneys, and colon. By eliminating accumulated toxins, these organs can perform their physiological roles more efficiently, thereby promoting systemic health and longevity.

3. **Immune System Support:** The immune system plays a pivotal role in defending the body against pathogens and maintaining homeostasis. Full body detoxification strengthens immune function by reducing the burden of toxins that can compromise immune responses. A robust immune system is better equipped to ward off infections and mitigate the risk of chronic diseases.

4. **Weight Management:** Toxins, particularly environmental pollutants and endocrine-disrupting chemicals, have been implicated in obesity and metabolic dysfunction. Full body detoxification aids in weight management by eliminating stored toxins that interfere with hormonal balance and metabolic regulation. Moreover, it can enhance nutrient absorption and facilitate the elimination of waste products, contributing to a healthy body composition.

5. **Radiant Skin and Youthful Appearance:** The skin serves as a major detoxification organ, eliminating toxins through sweat and sebum production. A full body detox can promote

clearer, more radiant skin by purging toxins that contribute to acne, inflammation, and premature aging. Furthermore, improved circulation and nutrient delivery to the skin can enhance its elasticity and youthful appearance.

6. **Mental Clarity and Emotional Well-being:** Toxins have been implicated in cognitive decline, mood disorders, and impaired mental function. By detoxifying the body, individuals often experience enhanced mental clarity, cognitive function, and emotional stability. Clearing the mind of toxic overload can foster a sense of inner peace, balance, and emotional resilience.

Conclusion

In conclusion, full body detoxification represents a holistic approach to health maintenance and disease prevention by eliminating accumulated toxins from the entire organism. Understanding the importance of full body detox is paramount in harnessing its therapeutic benefits and promoting overall well-being. By supporting vital organs, enhancing immune function, and rejuvenating cellular health, full body detox can pave the way for enhanced vitality, optimal health, and longevity. Embracing holistic detoxification practices can empower individuals to reclaim their health and vitality in an increasingly toxic world.

CHAPTER TWO

Preparing for Your Detox Journey: Mental and Physical Readiness

Embarking on a detox journey, whether it's a full body cleanse or a targeted program, requires careful preparation to ensure both mental resilience and physical readiness. Detoxification is not merely a physical process but also a mental and emotional endeavor that demands commitment, mindfulness, and self-awareness. In this discussion, we explore the essential steps to prepare yourself mentally and physically for a successful detox journey.

Understanding the Detox Process

Before diving into a detox program, it's crucial to have a clear understanding of the detox process and its potential effects on the body. Detoxification involves the mobilization and elimination of toxins accumulated in various tissues and organs. As toxins are released from storage sites, they may transiently enter the bloodstream, leading to detox symptoms such as headaches, fatigue, irritability, and digestive disturbances. These symptoms, often referred to as a "healing crisis" or "detox reaction," are a natural part of the cleansing process as the body purges accumulated toxins.

Setting Realistic Expectations

Setting realistic expectations is paramount to mental preparedness for a detox journey. It's essential to recognize that detoxification is not a quick fix or a one-size-fits-all solution. Results may vary depending on individual factors such as health status, lifestyle habits, and toxin exposure. Moreover, detoxification is not synonymous with weight loss, although some individuals may experience weight reduction as a byproduct of toxin elimination and improved metabolic function. By setting realistic goals and understanding that detox is a gradual, ongoing process, you can approach your journey with patience and perseverance.

Cultivating a Positive Mindset

A positive mindset is a powerful asset in navigating the challenges of a detox journey. Cultivate an attitude of self-compassion, acceptance, and non-judgment as you embark on this transformative process. Rather than viewing detox as a punitive measure or a deprivation diet, perceive it as an opportunity for self-care, renewal, and personal growth. Focus on the benefits of detoxification, such as increased energy, mental clarity, and overall well-being, to sustain motivation and momentum throughout your journey.

Embracing Self-Care Practices

Self-care plays a pivotal role in preparing for a detox journey, both mentally and physically. Prioritize activities that nourish your body, mind, and spirit, such as adequate sleep, regular exercise, stress management techniques, and mindfulness practices. Engage in activities that promote relaxation and rejuvenation, such as yoga, meditation, nature walks, and creative expression. Moreover, pay attention to your emotional needs and seek support from friends, family, or a professional counselor if needed. By nurturing yourself holistically, you lay a solid foundation for a successful detox experience.

Addressing Underlying Health Issues

Before embarking on a detox journey, it's essential to address any underlying health issues or medical conditions that may impact your ability to detoxify safely and effectively. Consult with a healthcare provider or qualified practitioner to assess your health status, discuss your goals and concerns, and determine the most appropriate detox approach for your individual needs. If you have pre-existing health conditions such as diabetes, cardiovascular disease, or autoimmune disorders, seek guidance from a healthcare professional who can tailor a detox protocol to accommodate your specific requirements.

Preparing Your Environment

Creating a supportive environment is crucial for a successful detox journey. Take proactive steps to minimize exposure to environmental toxins in your home, workplace, and personal care products. Opt for organic, whole foods whenever possible, and avoid processed foods, refined sugars, artificial additives, and inflammatory substances. Declutter your living space and create a tranquil sanctuary conducive to relaxation and rejuvenation. Surround yourself with positive influences, whether it's uplifting music, inspirational literature, or supportive friends who encourage and empower you on your journey.

Conclusion

Preparing for a detox journey involves both mental and physical readiness, encompassing a holistic approach to self-care and well-being. By understanding the detox process, setting realistic expectations, cultivating a positive mindset, embracing self-care practices, addressing underlying health issues, and preparing your environment, you can lay the groundwork for a transformative and empowering experience. Detoxification is not just about cleansing the body; it's about revitalizing the mind, nourishing the spirit, and reclaiming your innate capacity for health and vitality. Approach your detox journey with intention, mindfulness, and self-compassion, knowing that you have the power to enhance your well-being and thrive.

CHAPTER THREE

Meet Your Detox Guide: Dr. Barbara's Background and Expertise

As you embark on your detox journey, it's essential to have a knowledgeable and experienced guide to support you every step of the way. Meet Dr. Barbara, your trusted detox expert, who brings a wealth of expertise and a passion for holistic health to help you achieve your wellness goals. In this introduction, we delve into Dr. Barbara's background, qualifications, and areas of expertise, providing insight into her role as your dedicated detox guide.

Dr. Barbara's Educational Background

Dr. Barbara's journey into the field of holistic health and detoxification began with a solid foundation in traditional medicine. She obtained her medical degree from a prestigious institution, where she received comprehensive training in conventional diagnostics and treatment modalities. However, her quest for a deeper understanding of health and healing led her to explore complementary and alternative medicine modalities, including naturopathy, functional medicine, and integrative nutrition.

Driven by a desire to bridge the gap between conventional and holistic approaches to health, Dr. Barbara pursued additional training and certifications in various disciplines related to detoxification, nutrition, herbal medicine, and mind-body therapies. Her diverse educational background equips her with a broad spectrum of knowledge and tools to address the multifaceted aspects of detoxification and wellness.

Professional Experience and Clinical Practice

With over two decades of clinical experience, Dr. Barbara has dedicated her career to empowering individuals to reclaim their health and vitality through personalized, integrative approaches to wellness. She has worked in various clinical settings, including private practice, integrative health centers, and wellness retreats, where she has guided countless individuals on their journey to optimal health.

Dr. Barbara's clinical practice embodies a holistic approach that emphasizes the interconnectedness of mind, body, and spirit in achieving wellness. She takes a thorough and individualized approach to patient care, conducting comprehensive assessments, identifying underlying imbalances, and designing tailored treatment plans that address the root causes of health issues.

Areas of Expertise

Dr. Barbara's expertise encompasses a wide range of topics related to detoxification, holistic nutrition, herbal medicine, stress management, and lifestyle optimization. She specializes in guiding individuals through various detox protocols, including full body cleanses, liver detoxification, colon cleansing, and heavy metal detoxification.

In addition to her clinical work, Dr. Barbara is a passionate educator and advocate for holistic health, sharing her knowledge and expertise through workshops, seminars, online courses, and written publications. She believes in empowering individuals with the tools and knowledge they need to take charge of their health and make informed decisions that support their well-being.

Dr. Barbara's areas of expertise include:

1. **Detoxification Protocols:** Dr. Barbara is well-versed in designing safe and effective detox protocols tailored to individual needs, taking into account factors such as health status, toxin exposure, and lifestyle factors.

2. **Nutritional Counseling:** She provides personalized nutritional counseling to optimize diet and lifestyle choices, with a focus on whole foods, plant-based nutrition, and targeted supplementation to support detoxification pathways.

3. **Herbal Medicine:** Dr. Barbara utilizes the healing power of herbs and botanicals to support detoxification, enhance liver function, promote digestion, and balance the body's natural rhythms.

4. **Mind-Body Medicine:** She incorporates mind-body techniques such as meditation, breathwork, yoga, and stress management strategies to promote relaxation, resilience, and emotional well-being during the detox process.

Conclusion

In conclusion, Dr. Barbara is your dedicated detox guide, bringing a wealth of knowledge, experience, and expertise to support you on your wellness journey. With a solid foundation in traditional medicine and a passion for holistic health, she combines the best of both worlds to offer personalized, integrative approaches to detoxification and wellness. Whether you're embarking on a full body cleanse, addressing specific health concerns, or seeking to optimize your lifestyle for vibrant health, Dr. Barbara is committed to empowering you with the tools and support you need to thrive.

CHAPTER FOUR

The Science Behind Detoxification: How It Benefits Your Body

Detoxification, often touted as a cornerstone of holistic health practices, is grounded in scientific principles that elucidate its profound benefits for the body. Far from being a fad or trendy buzzword, detoxification encompasses a complex series of biochemical processes orchestrated by the body's innate detoxification pathways. In this exploration, we delve into the science behind detoxification, elucidating how it benefits the body at the cellular, biochemical, and systemic levels.

Understanding Detoxification Pathways

Detoxification is a multifaceted process that occurs primarily in the liver, but also involves other organs such as the kidneys, colon, skin, and lymphatic system. At its core, detoxification entails the conversion of fat-soluble toxins into water-soluble compounds that can be eliminated from the body via urine, feces, sweat, and respiration. This process involves a series of enzymatic reactions mediated by specialized enzymes known as cytochrome P450 enzymes, as well as phase II conjugation enzymes such as glutathione, glucuronidation, and sulfation enzymes.

Liver Detoxification

The liver plays a central role in detoxification, serving as the body's primary detox organ. It performs two phases of detoxification: Phase I and Phase II. In Phase I, fat-soluble toxins are metabolized into intermediate compounds through oxidation, reduction, and hydrolysis reactions, rendering them more water-soluble but potentially more reactive and toxic in the process. Phase II involves conjugation reactions, where these intermediate compounds are bound to water-soluble molecules such as glutathione, glucuronic acid, and sulfate, facilitating their excretion from the body.

Key Players in Detoxification

Several key players are involved in the detoxification process, including:

1. **Antioxidants:** Antioxidants such as glutathione, vitamin C, vitamin E, and selenium play a crucial role in neutralizing free radicals and oxidative stress generated during detoxification. They protect cells from damage and support the regeneration of detox enzymes.

2. **Nutrients:** Essential nutrients such as B vitamins, magnesium, zinc, and amino acids are cofactors required for the optimal function of detox enzymes. Adequate nutrient intake is essential for maintaining the integrity and efficiency of detoxification pathways.

3. **Hydration:** Adequate hydration is vital for supporting detoxification by facilitating the elimination of water-soluble toxins through urine and promoting optimal kidney function. Drinking plenty of water helps flush toxins out of the body and maintains fluid balance.

4. **Fiber:** Dietary fiber plays a critical role in detoxification by promoting regular bowel movements and preventing the reabsorption of toxins in the colon. Fiber-rich foods such as fruits, vegetables, whole grains, and legumes support optimal digestive function and elimination.

Benefits of Detoxification

Detoxification confers a myriad of benefits for the body, including:

1. **Improved Liver Function:** By supporting liver detoxification pathways, detoxification enhances the liver's ability to metabolize and eliminate toxins efficiently, thereby promoting optimal liver function and reducing the risk of liver diseases.

2. **Enhanced Cellular Health:** Detoxification helps rid the body of accumulated toxins that can impair cellular function, compromise mitochondrial health, and contribute to oxidative stress and inflammation. By promoting cellular detoxification, it supports overall cellular health and longevity.

3. **Reduced Oxidative Stress:** Oxidative stress, resulting from an imbalance between free radicals and antioxidants, is implicated in various chronic diseases and aging processes. Detoxification helps mitigate oxidative stress by neutralizing free radicals and enhancing antioxidant defenses, thereby reducing the risk of oxidative damage to cells and tissues.

4. **Balanced Hormones:** Toxins, particularly endocrine-disrupting chemicals, can interfere with hormonal balance and disrupt endocrine function. Detoxification supports hormonal equilibrium by eliminating hormone-disrupting toxins and promoting optimal endocrine function.

5. **Enhanced Immune Function:** A healthy immune system is essential for defending the body against pathogens and maintaining overall health. Detoxification supports immune function by reducing the burden of toxins that can compromise immune responses and impair immune function.

6. **Increased Energy and Vitality:** By eliminating toxins and metabolic waste products, detoxification enhances energy production, cellular metabolism, and mitochondrial function, leading to increased energy levels, vitality, and overall well-being.

Conclusion

In conclusion, the science behind detoxification elucidates its profound benefits for the body, ranging from improved liver function and enhanced cellular health to reduced oxidative stress and balanced hormones. Detoxification is a complex biochemical process orchestrated by the body's innate detoxification pathways, involving enzymatic reactions, antioxidant defenses, and nutrient cofactors. By supporting detoxification through proper nutrition, hydration, and lifestyle practices, individuals can optimize their body's ability to eliminate toxins and promote overall health and vitality. Embracing detoxification as a foundational aspect of holistic health and wellness empowers individuals to reclaim their health, prevent disease, and thrive in an increasingly toxic world.

CHAPTER FIVE

Day 1-7: Cleansing Phase - Removing Toxins from Your System

The cleansing phase, spanning the first seven days of your detox journey, marks the initiation of toxin removal from your system. During this pivotal period, your body undergoes a series of physiological adjustments to facilitate the elimination of accumulated toxins and metabolic waste products. Here's a detailed overview of what to expect during the cleansing phase and strategies to optimize detoxification for optimal results.

Understanding the Cleansing Phase

1. **Activation of Detox Pathways:** As you commence your detox journey, your body initiates the activation of detoxification pathways, particularly in the liver, kidneys, colon, and skin. Enzymatic reactions involved in Phase I and Phase II detoxification are upregulated, enhancing the metabolism and elimination of toxins from various tissues and organs.

2. **Mobilization of Stored Toxins:** During the cleansing phase, stored toxins trapped in adipose tissue, organs, and cellular compartments are mobilized for elimination. This process may lead to transient symptoms such as headaches, fatigue, irritability, and digestive disturbances as toxins are released into circulation for excretion.

3. **Supporting Organs of Elimination:** The liver, kidneys, colon, lungs, and skin play pivotal roles in eliminating toxins from the body. Adequate hydration, dietary fiber, and lymphatic support are essential for optimizing the function of these organs and facilitating the efficient removal of toxins through urine, feces, sweat, and respiration.

Strategies for Optimal Detoxification

1. **Hydration:** Drink plenty of water throughout the day to support hydration and facilitate the elimination of water-soluble toxins through urine. Aim for at least 8-10 glasses of filtered water daily, and consider incorporating herbal teas and electrolyte-rich beverages to replenish minerals lost through detoxification.

2. **Nutrient-Dense Diet:** Focus on consuming nutrient-dense, whole foods that support detoxification and provide essential nutrients required for optimal organ function. Emphasize a plant-based diet rich in fruits, vegetables, leafy greens, whole grains, legumes, nuts, and seeds, while minimizing processed foods, refined sugars, artificial additives, and inflammatory substances.

3. **Liver Support:** Incorporate liver-supportive foods and herbs into your diet, such as cruciferous vegetables (e.g., broccoli, kale, cabbage), beets, dandelion greens, artichokes, garlic, turmeric, milk thistle, and dandelion root. These foods

contain compounds that enhance liver detoxification pathways and promote bile flow, facilitating the elimination of toxins.

4. **Colon Cleansing:** Support colon health and regular bowel movements by consuming fiber-rich foods, staying hydrated, and incorporating natural laxatives such as psyllium husk, flaxseeds, chia seeds, and magnesium citrate. Colon cleansing promotes the elimination of waste products and prevents the reabsorption of toxins in the colon.

5. **Sweat Therapy:** Incorporate sweat-inducing activities such as sauna sessions, hot baths, steam baths, and vigorous exercise to promote sweating and facilitate the elimination of toxins through the skin. Sweating enhances lymphatic circulation, promotes detoxification, and supports overall well-being.

6. **Rest and Relaxation:** Prioritize restorative practices such as meditation, deep breathing exercises, gentle yoga, and adequate sleep to support the body's detoxification processes and reduce stress levels. Stress reduction is essential for optimal detoxification, as chronic stress can impair immune function and detoxification pathways.

Conclusion

The cleansing phase, spanning the first seven days of your detox journey, is a critical period for removing toxins from your system and initiating physiological adjustments to support detoxification. By implementing strategies such as hydration, nutrient-dense nutrition, liver support, colon cleansing, sweat therapy, and stress reduction, you can optimize detoxification and promote overall health and vitality. Embrace this transformative phase with intention, mindfulness, and self-care, knowing that you're taking proactive steps to rejuvenate your body and reclaim your well-being.

CHAPTER SIX

Day 8-14: Rejuvenation Phase - Replenishing Nutrients and Energy

As you transition from the cleansing phase into the rejuvenation phase of your detox journey, the focus shifts from toxin removal to replenishing nutrients, restoring energy levels, and supporting overall vitality. During this critical period, your body undergoes a process of renewal and regeneration, harnessing the restorative power of wholesome nutrition, targeted supplementation, and rejuvenating practices. Here's a comprehensive guide to navigating the rejuvenation phase effectively and optimizing your body's capacity for healing and revitalization.

Key Objectives of the Rejuvenation Phase

1. **Nutrient Repletion:** Replenish essential nutrients, vitamins, minerals, and antioxidants depleted during the cleansing phase to support cellular repair, metabolic function, and overall well-being.

2. **Energy Restoration:** Restore energy levels, vitality, and stamina by providing the body with nourishing foods, hydration, and restorative practices that promote optimal energy production and mitochondrial function.

3. **Cellular Repair:** Support cellular repair and regeneration by providing the body with the building blocks necessary for tissue renewal, DNA synthesis, and protein synthesis.

4. **Balanced Blood Sugar:** Stabilize blood sugar levels and prevent energy fluctuations by consuming balanced meals and snacks that combine complex carbohydrates, healthy fats, and lean proteins.

Strategies for Rejuvenation

1. **Wholesome Nutrition:** Emphasize a nutrient-dense, whole foods-based diet rich in fruits, vegetables, leafy greens, whole grains, legumes, nuts, seeds, and lean proteins. Incorporate a variety of colorful fruits and vegetables to maximize antioxidant intake and support cellular health.

2. **Hydration:** Continue to prioritize hydration by drinking plenty of water, herbal teas, and electrolyte-rich beverages throughout the day. Hydration supports detoxification, cellular function, and metabolic processes, promoting overall vitality and well-being.

3. **Supplementation:** Consider incorporating targeted supplements to support detoxification, cellular repair, and energy production. Key supplements may include omega-3 fatty acids, probiotics, vitamin D, magnesium, B-complex vitamins, antioxidants (e.g., vitamin C, vitamin E, selenium),

and adaptogenic herbs (e.g., ashwagandha, rhodiola, holy basil) to support stress resilience and adrenal function.

4. **Balanced Meals:** Plan balanced meals and snacks that provide a combination of complex carbohydrates, healthy fats, and lean proteins to stabilize blood sugar levels and sustain energy throughout the day. Aim for nutrient-rich foods that nourish the body and support optimal metabolic function.

5. **Restorative Practices:** Incorporate restorative practices such as meditation, deep breathing exercises, gentle yoga, and massage therapy to promote relaxation, reduce stress levels, and support overall well-being. Prioritize self-care activities that nurture your body, mind, and spirit during this rejuvenation phase.

6. **Physical Activity:** Engage in moderate physical activity such as walking, cycling, swimming, or yoga to promote circulation, enhance mood, and support detoxification. Choose activities that you enjoy and listen to your body's cues to avoid overexertion.

7. **Sleep Quality:** Prioritize quality sleep by establishing a consistent sleep schedule, creating a restful sleep environment, and practicing relaxation techniques before bedtime. Adequate sleep is essential for cellular repair, hormone balance, and overall health and vitality.

Conclusion

The rejuvenation phase, spanning days 8-14 of your detox journey, offers an opportunity for replenishing nutrients, restoring energy levels, and supporting overall vitality. By implementing strategies such as wholesome nutrition, hydration, supplementation, balanced meals, restorative practices, physical activity, and quality sleep, you can optimize your body's capacity for healing and revitalization. Embrace this phase with gratitude and intention, knowing that you're nurturing your body and supporting its innate capacity for health and well-being.

CHAPTER SEVEN

Day 15-21: Transformation Phase - Integrating Healthy Habits for Long-Term Wellness

As you enter the transformation phase of your detox journey, spanning days 15-21, the focus shifts towards integrating healthy habits and sustainable lifestyle changes that promote long-term wellness. This phase represents a pivotal opportunity to consolidate the gains achieved during the cleansing and rejuvenation phases and lay the foundation for a healthier, more vibrant future. Here's a comprehensive guide to navigating the transformation phase effectively and embracing lifelong habits that support optimal health and well-being.

Key Objectives of the Transformation Phase

1. **Behavioral Change:** Cultivate new habits and behaviors that support your health and wellness goals, such as mindful eating, regular physical activity, stress management, and self-care practices.

2. **Mind-Body Connection:** Deepen your awareness of the mind-body connection and incorporate practices that promote mental, emotional, and spiritual well-being, such as meditation, yoga, gratitude journaling, and creative expression.

3. **Nutrition Optimization:** Fine-tune your dietary choices to prioritize whole, nutrient-dense foods that nourish your body, support detoxification, and promote optimal metabolic function.

4. **Lifestyle Alignment:** Align your lifestyle with your health goals by optimizing sleep quality, managing stress levels, fostering supportive relationships, and creating a balanced routine that prioritizes self-care and well-being.

Strategies for Transformation

1. **Mindful Eating:** Practice mindful eating by paying attention to hunger cues, savoring each bite, and tuning into your body's signals of hunger and satiety. Choose whole, minimally processed foods that nourish your body and support optimal health.

2. **Meal Planning:** Plan and prepare balanced meals and snacks ahead of time to ensure that you have nutritious options readily available. Incorporate a variety of fruits, vegetables, whole grains, lean proteins, and healthy fats into your meals to maximize nutrient intake.

3. **Portion Control:** Practice portion control by listening to your body's hunger and fullness signals and avoiding oversized portions. Use smaller plates, bowls, and utensils to help regulate portion sizes and prevent overeating.

4. **Regular Physical Activity:** Make physical activity a regular part of your routine by engaging in activities that you enjoy, such as walking, jogging, cycling, swimming, dancing, or yoga. Aim for at least 30 minutes of moderate-intensity exercise most days of the week to support cardiovascular health, muscle strength, and overall well-being.

5. **Stress Management:** Incorporate stress management techniques such as meditation, deep breathing exercises, progressive muscle relaxation, and mindfulness practices into your daily routine to promote relaxation, reduce stress levels, and enhance resilience.

6. **Social Support:** Surround yourself with supportive friends, family members, or community groups who share your health and wellness goals. Seek out social connections that uplift and inspire you, and engage in activities that foster a sense of belonging and connection.

7. **Self-Care Practices:** Prioritize self-care practices that nurture your body, mind, and spirit, such as taking regular breaks, spending time in nature, indulging in hobbies, and practicing gratitude. Schedule time for relaxation and rejuvenation to recharge your batteries and maintain balance in your life.

8. **Continuous Learning:** Stay informed about the latest developments in health and wellness research, and continue to educate yourself about topics that interest you. Take

courses, attend workshops, and read books or articles that expand your knowledge and deepen your understanding of holistic health practices.

Conclusion

The transformation phase, spanning days 15-21 of your detox journey, represents a pivotal period for integrating healthy habits and sustainable lifestyle changes that promote long-term wellness. By focusing on behavioral change, mind-body connection, nutrition optimization, and lifestyle alignment, you can cultivate a foundation of health and vitality that supports your well-being for years to come. Embrace this phase with enthusiasm and commitment, knowing that you have the power to transform your health and create a life of abundance, vitality, and joy.

CHAPTER EIGHT

Essential Foods for Detox: Exploring Nutrient-Rich I€ngredients

Incorporating nutrient-rich foods into your diet is essential for supporting the body's natural detoxification processes and promoting overall health and vitality. By focusing on whole, minimally processed foods that are rich in vitamins, minerals, antioxidants, and phytonutrients, you can nourish your body and optimize its ability to eliminate toxins and restore balance. In this exploration, we delve into essential foods for detox, highlighting their detoxifying properties and health benefits.

1. Leafy Greens

Leafy greens such as kale, spinach, Swiss chard, collard greens, and arugula are nutritional powerhouses packed with vitamins, minerals, and antioxidants. They are rich in chlorophyll, a natural detoxifier that helps eliminate toxins from the body and supports liver function. Leafy greens also contain fiber, which promotes regular bowel movements and aids in the removal of waste products and toxins from the colon.

2. Cruciferous Vegetables

Cruciferous vegetables, including broccoli, cauliflower, Brussels sprouts, cabbage, and bok choy, are renowned for their detoxifying properties. They contain compounds called glucosinolates, which are converted into sulforaphane and indole-3-carbinol during digestion. These compounds support liver detoxification pathways, enhance the elimination of toxins, and reduce the risk of chronic diseases such as cancer and cardiovascular disease.

3. Berries

Berries such as blueberries, strawberries, raspberries, and blackberries are rich in antioxidants, including flavonoids, anthocyanins, and vitamin C. These antioxidants help neutralize free radicals, reduce oxidative stress, and protect cells from damage caused by environmental toxins and pollutants. Berries also contain fiber, which supports digestive health and promotes the elimination of toxins from the body.

4. Citrus Fruits

Citrus fruits such as lemons, limes, oranges, and grapefruits are excellent sources of vitamin C, a potent antioxidant that supports immune function and enhances detoxification. Citrus fruits also contain limonoids and flavonoids, which have been shown to promote liver health, stimulate the production of detox enzymes, and facilitate the elimination of toxins from the body.

5. Garlic

Garlic is renowned for its numerous health benefits, including its ability to support detoxification and immune function. It contains sulfur compounds such as allicin, which have anti-inflammatory, antimicrobial, and detoxifying properties. Garlic also supports liver detoxification pathways, enhances circulation, and promotes cardiovascular health.

6. Turmeric

Turmeric is a golden-yellow spice derived from the Curcuma longa plant, prized for its anti-inflammatory and antioxidant properties. It contains curcumin, a bioactive compound that supports liver function, reduces inflammation, and enhances detoxification. Turmeric also stimulates bile production, which aids in the digestion and absorption of fats and supports the elimination of toxins from the body.

7. Ginger

Ginger is a versatile root with potent anti-inflammatory and antioxidant properties. It contains bioactive compounds such as gingerol and shogaols, which support digestive health, reduce inflammation, and enhance detoxification. Ginger also stimulates circulation, promotes sweating, and aids in the elimination of toxins through the skin.

8. Green Tea

Green tea is rich in catechins, a type of antioxidant that has been shown to support detoxification, boost metabolism, and promote weight loss. It also contains theanine, an amino acid that promotes relaxation and reduces stress, which can support overall well-being during the detox process.

Conclusion

Incorporating nutrient-rich foods such as leafy greens, cruciferous vegetables, berries, citrus fruits, garlic, turmeric, ginger, and green tea into your diet is essential for supporting detoxification and promoting overall health and vitality. These foods are packed with vitamins, minerals, antioxidants, and phytonutrients that help neutralize free radicals, reduce inflammation, support liver function, and enhance the elimination of toxins from the body. By making these foods a staple of your diet, you can nourish your body and support its natural detoxification processes for optimal health and well-being.

CHAPTER NINE

Creating detox-friendly recipes tailored to each phase of your detox journey can enhance the effectiveness of your cleanse while ensuring you're nourished and satisfied throughout the process. Here are meal plans and ideas for each phase:

Cleansing Phase (Day 1-7):

Breakfast:

- Green smoothie with spinach, kale, cucumber, celery, lemon juice, and a splash of coconut water.

- Chia seed pudding topped with berries and a sprinkle of cinnamon.

Lunch:

- Quinoa salad with mixed greens, cherry tomatoes, cucumbers, avocado, and a lemon-tahini dressing.

- Detox vegetable soup made with broth, carrots, celery, onions, kale, and garlic.

Dinner:

- Baked salmon with steamed asparagus and roasted Brussels sprouts.

- Stir-fried tofu with broccoli, bell peppers, and snap peas in a ginger-garlic sauce.

Snacks:

- Sliced cucumber with hummus.

- Raw almonds and walnuts.

- Apple slices with almond butter.

Rejuvenation Phase (Day 8-14):

Breakfast:

- Overnight oats with almond milk, sliced banana, walnuts, and a drizzle of honey.

- Greek yogurt parfait with mixed berries, granola, and a dollop of honey.

Lunch:

- Grilled chicken salad with mixed greens, roasted beets, goat cheese, and balsamic vinaigrette.

- Lentil and vegetable stir-fry with brown rice and a side of steamed broccoli.

Dinner:

- Baked cod with roasted sweet potatoes and sautéed spinach.

- Zucchini noodles with marinara sauce and grilled shrimp.

Snacks:

- Carrot sticks with tzatziki dip.

- Trail mix with dried fruit and pumpkin seeds.

- Sliced pear with ricotta cheese and a drizzle of honey.

Transformation Phase (Day 15-21):

Breakfast:

- Avocado toast on whole grain bread with sliced tomatoes and a sprinkle of hemp seeds.

- Vegetable omelet with bell peppers, onions, spinach, and feta cheese.

Lunch:

- Quinoa Buddha bowl with roasted vegetables, chickpeas, avocado, and tahini dressing.

- Turkey and avocado wrap with lettuce, tomato, and whole grain tortilla.

Dinner:

- Grilled steak with roasted cauliflower and a mixed green salad.

- Spaghetti squash with marinara sauce and turkey meatballs.

Snacks:

- Edamame with sea salt.

- Greek yogurt with honey and sliced almonds.

- Rice cakes with mashed avocado and cherry tomatoes.

Conclusion: These meal plans and recipe ideas provide a variety of delicious and nutritious options to support each phase of your detox journey. By focusing on whole, nutrient-rich foods and incorporating a balance of lean proteins, healthy fats, fiber, and antioxidant-rich fruits and vegetables, you can optimize your detox experience while nourishing your body and promoting long-term wellness. Adjust portion sizes and ingredients based on your individual preferences and dietary restrictions, and remember to listen to your body's hunger and fullness cues throughout the process.

CHAPTER TEN

Maintaining Your Results: Tips for Sustaining a Healthy Lifestyle After the Detox

Completing a detox program is a significant achievement, but the real challenge lies in maintaining your results and transitioning to a sustainable, long-term healthy lifestyle. To ensure that the benefits of your detox are lasting, it's essential to incorporate healthy habits and mindful practices into your daily routine. Here are some tips for sustaining a healthy lifestyle after the detox:

1. Embrace Whole Foods: Focus on consuming a diet rich in whole, minimally processed foods such as fruits, vegetables, whole grains, lean proteins, and healthy fats. These nutrient-dense foods provide essential vitamins, minerals, antioxidants, and fiber to support overall health and well-being.

2. Practice Portion Control: Be mindful of portion sizes and listen to your body's hunger and fullness cues. Avoid overeating and practice mindful eating by savoring each bite, chewing slowly, and paying attention to your body's signals of hunger and satiety.

3. Stay Hydrated: Drink plenty of water throughout the day to stay hydrated and support detoxification. Aim for at least 8-10 glasses of water daily, and consider incorporating herbal teas, infused water, and electrolyte-rich beverages to stay hydrated and replenish fluids.

4. Prioritize Physical Activity: Make regular physical activity a priority by incorporating exercise into your daily routine. Choose activities that you enjoy, such as walking, jogging, swimming, cycling, yoga, or dancing, and aim for at least 30 minutes of moderate-intensity exercise most days of the week.

5. Manage Stress: Practice stress management techniques such as meditation, deep breathing exercises, progressive muscle relaxation, and mindfulness practices to reduce stress levels and promote relaxation. Prioritize self-care activities that nurture your body, mind, and spirit and help you cope with stress more effectively.

6. Get Adequate Sleep: Prioritize quality sleep by establishing a consistent sleep schedule, creating a restful sleep environment, and practicing relaxation techniques before bedtime. Aim for 7-9 hours of sleep per night to support overall health, cognitive function, and well-being.

7. Cultivate Healthy Habits: Incorporate healthy habits into your daily routine, such as meal planning, grocery shopping, cooking at home, and packing nutritious snacks. Create a supportive environment that fosters healthy choices and encourages positive behaviors.

8. Practice Mindful Eating: Be mindful of what you eat, how you eat, and why you eat. Pay attention to hunger and fullness cues, eat slowly, and savor each bite. Avoid distractions such as screens or multitasking while eating, and cultivate a deeper appreciation for the flavors and textures of your food.

9. Stay Connected: Surround yourself with supportive friends, family members, or community groups who share your health and wellness goals. Seek out social connections that uplift and inspire you, and engage in activities that foster a sense of belonging and connection.

10. Be Flexible and Forgiving: Remember that maintaining a healthy lifestyle is not about perfection but about progress. Be kind to yourself, and don't be too hard on yourself if you slip up or have setbacks. Focus on making small, sustainable changes over time, and celebrate your successes along the way.

By incorporating these tips into your daily life, you can sustain the benefits of your detox program and continue to thrive in the long term. Remember that maintaining a healthy lifestyle is a journey, not a destination, and every positive choice you make contributes to your overall well-being and vitality.

BONUS: SOME HERBAL AND HOLISTIC APPROACHES TO KNOW

Acupuncture:

Definition: Acupuncture is a traditional Chinese medicine practice that involves inserting thin needles into specific points on the body. It's believed to stimulate energy flow, known as qi (pronounced "chee"), and restore balance to the body's systems. It's used to alleviate pain, treat various health conditions, and promote overall wellness.

Ingredients: The ingredients for acupuncture are minimal and primarily involve thin, sterile needles made of stainless steel or other materials.

How to Prepare: Preparing for acupuncture involves ensuring that the needles and the environment are sterile. Practitioners may also conduct a thorough assessment of the patient's health history and current condition to determine the appropriate acupuncture points to target.

Dosage: There isn't a fixed dosage for acupuncture as it varies depending on the condition being treated, the individual's health status, and the practitioner's assessment. Acupuncture sessions may range from a single treatment to multiple sessions over several weeks or months.

How to Use: During an acupuncture session, the practitioner inserts needles into specific points on the body, typically leaving them in place for around 15 to 30 minutes. The needles may be manipulated manually or stimulated with heat or electricity to enhance the therapeutic effect. Some practitioners may also recommend complementary therapies such as herbal supplements or dietary changes to support the acupuncture treatment.

Side Effects: Common side effects of acupuncture are minimal and may include temporary soreness, bruising, or bleeding at the needle insertion sites. In rare cases, more serious side effects such as infection or organ injury may occur, especially if proper sterile procedures are not followed or if the practitioner lacks adequate training. It's essential to seek acupuncture treatment from a qualified and licensed practitioner to minimize risks. Additionally, acupuncture may not be suitable for everyone, particularly those with certain medical conditions or who are pregnant, so it's important to consult with a healthcare provider before undergoing treatment.

Aloe Vera Juice:

Definition: Aloe vera juice is a liquid extracted from the aloe vera plant, known for its medicinal properties and health benefits. It's commonly consumed for its purported digestive, skin-healing, and immune-boosting properties.

Ingredients: Aloe vera juice is primarily composed of the gel-like substance found in the inner leaf of the aloe vera plant. Some commercial preparations may also contain added ingredients such as preservatives, flavorings, or sweeteners.

How to Prepare: Aloe vera juice is typically extracted from the inner fillet of the aloe vera leaf. The leaf is cut open, and the gel is scooped out and blended into a liquid. Commercially available aloe vera juice undergoes processing and may involve filtration and pasteurization to ensure safety and stability.

Dosage: The recommended dosage of aloe vera juice can vary depending on the individual's health goals and tolerance. It's advisable to start with a small amount, such as 1 to 2 ounces per day, and gradually increase as needed. It's essential to follow the manufacturer's instructions or consult with a healthcare provider for personalized guidance.

How to Use: Aloe vera juice can be consumed on its own or mixed with other beverages such as water or juice. Some people prefer to drink it first thing in the morning or before meals to support digestion. It can also be used topically to soothe skin irritation or sunburn.

Side Effects: While aloe vera juice is generally considered safe for most people when consumed in moderation, excessive intake may cause digestive upset, such as diarrhea or abdominal cramping, due to its laxative properties. Long-term use of high doses of aloe vera juice has been associated with potential adverse effects on the liver and kidneys. Individuals with underlying health conditions, such as diabetes or kidney disease, should use aloe vera juice with caution and consult with a healthcare provider before starting regular consumption. Additionally, some people may experience allergic reactions or skin irritation from topical application of aloe vera juice, so it's advisable to perform a patch test before using it extensively.

Bentonite Clay:

Definition: Bentonite clay is a natural clay formed from volcanic ash deposits and is known for its absorbent properties. It's commonly used in skincare, detoxification, and as a digestive supplement.

Ingredients: Bentonite clay is composed primarily of volcanic ash and minerals such as calcium, magnesium, and silica. It's available in powder form.

How to Prepare: To prepare bentonite clay for topical use, mix it with water or other liquid to form a paste. For internal use, it can be mixed with water or added to food or beverages.

Dosage: The dosage of bentonite clay varies depending on its intended use. For internal use, typical doses range from 1 teaspoon to 1 tablespoon mixed with water once or twice daily.

It's essential to drink plenty of water when consuming bentonite clay to prevent dehydration and constipation.

How to Use: For skincare, bentonite clay can be applied as a mask to the face or body to absorb excess oil and impurities. It's left on for a few minutes to dry before rinsing off with warm water. Internally, bentonite clay is used as a dietary supplement to support detoxification and digestive health.

Side Effects: While bentonite clay is generally considered safe for topical and internal use, some people may experience mild side effects such as stomach upset or constipation. It's essential to start with a small dose and monitor for any adverse reactions. Long-term or excessive use of bentonite clay internally may lead to mineral deficiencies or bowel obstruction. Pregnant or breastfeeding women and individuals with certain medical conditions should consult with a healthcare provider before using bentonite clay.

Charcoal Detox:

Definition: Charcoal detox refers to the use of activated charcoal, typically derived from sources like coconut shells or bamboo, to help remove toxins and impurities from the body. Activated charcoal is known for its highly porous surface, which allows it to trap toxins and chemicals.

Ingredients: Activated charcoal is the primary ingredient used in charcoal detox. It's available in various forms, including powder, capsules, and tablets.

How to Prepare: Preparing for a charcoal detox involves selecting the appropriate form of activated charcoal and following the recommended dosage instructions provided on the product packaging or as directed by a healthcare provider.

Dosage: The dosage of activated charcoal for detoxification purposes varies depending on factors such as the individual's weight, age, and overall health status. It's essential to follow the recommended dosage instructions carefully to avoid potential side effects.

How to Use: Activated charcoal can be consumed orally by mixing it with water or other liquids, or it may be taken in capsule or tablet form. It's typically taken on an empty stomach, either between meals or several hours before or after eating, to maximize its detoxifying effects. Activated charcoal can also be used topically in skincare products to absorb excess oil and impurities from the skin.

Side Effects: While activated charcoal is generally considered safe for short-term use, it may cause side effects such as constipation, black stools, or gastrointestinal discomfort in some individuals. It's essential to drink plenty of water when consuming activated charcoal to prevent dehydration and ensure proper elimination of toxins from the body. Activated charcoal may also interfere with the absorption of certain medications, so it's advisable to take it at least two hours before or after taking any medications. Individuals with gastrointestinal conditions, such as blockages or bleeding, should avoid using activated charcoal without consulting with a healthcare provider.

Chlorella Supplements:

Definition: Chlorella supplements are derived from a type of single-celled green algae called Chlorella vulgaris. They are known for their high nutrient content, including vitamins, minerals, antioxidants, and amino acids.

Ingredients: Chlorella supplements contain dried and processed Chlorella vulgaris algae. They may be available in various forms, including tablets, capsules, powders, and liquid extracts.

How to Prepare: Preparing for chlorella supplementation involves selecting the desired form of the supplement and following the recommended dosage instructions provided on the product packaging or as advised by a healthcare provider.

Dosage: The dosage of chlorella supplements varies depending on factors such as the individual's age, weight, and health goals. It's essential to follow the recommended dosage instructions to ensure safety and effectiveness.

How to Use: Chlorella supplements can be consumed orally by swallowing tablets or capsules with water, or they may be mixed into smoothies, juices, or other beverages. Some people also use chlorella powder to sprinkle on food or incorporate into recipes. Chlorella supplements are typically taken once or twice daily with meals.

Side Effects: Chlorella supplements are generally well-tolerated by most people when taken in recommended doses. However, some individuals may experience mild side effects such as digestive upset, including nausea, diarrhea, or flatulence. These side effects are usually temporary and subside with continued use or by adjusting the dosage. Chlorella supplements may also cause allergic reactions in some individuals, particularly those with sensitivities to algae or seafood. It's advisable to start with a low dose and monitor for any adverse reactions. Individuals with certain medical conditions or who are pregnant or breastfeeding should consult with a healthcare provider before starting chlorella supplementation.

Colon Cleansing:

Definition: Colon cleansing, also known as colonic irrigation or colon hydrotherapy, is a practice aimed at removing toxins and waste buildup from the colon. It typically involves flushing the colon with water or other substances to stimulate bowel movements and promote detoxification.

Ingredients: Colon cleansing procedures may use various ingredients, including water, herbal solutions, saline solutions, or other substances designed to soften stool and facilitate elimination.

How to Prepare: Preparing for a colon cleansing procedure may involve dietary restrictions, such as avoiding solid foods for a period before the procedure, and ensuring proper hydration. It's essential to follow any instructions provided by the healthcare provider or practitioner performing the colon cleansing.

Dosage: The frequency and duration of colon cleansing procedures vary depending on factors such as individual health goals and the specific method used. Some people may undergo colon cleansing as a one-time treatment, while others may incorporate it into a regular detoxification regimen.

How to Use: Colon cleansing procedures may be performed by healthcare professionals in clinical settings or by using at-home kits. During the procedure, a tube is inserted into the rectum, and water or a cleansing solution is gently introduced into the colon to flush out waste material. The process typically takes about 45 minutes to an hour.

Side Effects: While colon cleansing may offer temporary relief from symptoms such as constipation or bloating, it's important to note that it's not necessary for everyone and may carry risks. Potential side effects of colon cleansing include dehydration, electrolyte imbalance, perforation of the colon, infection, and disruption of the natural balance of bacteria in the gut. Colon cleansing may also interfere with the body's natural bowel function and lead to dependence on laxatives for regular bowel movements. Individuals considering colon cleansing should consult with a healthcare provider to weigh the potential benefits and risks.

Cranberry Juice:

Definition: Cranberry juice is a tart and tangy beverage made from the juice of cranberries, which are small, red berries known for their high antioxidant content and potential health benefits.

Ingredients: Cranberry juice is made primarily from cranberries, which contain vitamins, minerals, antioxidants, and phytonutrients such as flavonoids and polyphenols.

How to Prepare: Commercially available cranberry juice is typically prepared by pressing or crushing cranberries to extract the juice, which may be further processed and filtered to remove pulp and solids. Some varieties of cranberry juice may contain added sugars or other ingredients for flavor enhancement.

Dosage: There isn't a specific dosage for cranberry juice, but incorporating it into your diet in moderation can provide potential health benefits. Drinking one to two glasses of cranberry juice per day is often recommended for urinary tract health.

How to Use: Cranberry juice can be consumed on its own as a refreshing beverage or mixed with other juices or water. Some people also use cranberry juice as an ingredient in cocktails, smoothies, or salad dressings. It's essential to choose unsweetened cranberry juice or opt for varieties with minimal added sugars to maximize the health benefits.

Side Effects: While cranberry juice is generally safe for most people when consumed in moderation, some individuals may experience side effects such as gastrointestinal upset or diarrhea, particularly if consumed in large quantities. Cranberry juice may also interact with certain medications, such as blood thinners, and individuals with a history of kidney stones may need to limit their intake due to the high oxalate content of cranberries. It's advisable to consult with a healthcare provider before incorporating cranberry juice into your diet, especially if you have underlying health conditions or are taking medications.

Detox Baths:

Definition: Detox baths are a form of hydrotherapy that involves soaking in a bath containing various ingredients believed to help remove toxins from the body, promote relaxation, and support overall well-being.

Ingredients: Detox baths may include a variety of ingredients such as Epsom salts, baking soda, essential oils, apple cider vinegar, bentonite clay, ginger, and herbs like lavender or chamomile.

How to Prepare: Preparing a detox bath involves adding the desired ingredients to a bathtub filled with warm water. The water temperature should be comfortable for soaking, and the ingredients should be thoroughly mixed into the water to ensure even distribution.

Dosage: There isn't a specific dosage for detox baths, as the frequency and duration of soaking can vary depending on individual preferences and needs. Some people may enjoy a detox bath once a week as part of their self-care routine, while others may choose to soak more or less frequently.

How to Use: To use a detox bath, simply immerse yourself in the tub and soak for 20 to 30 minutes or longer, allowing the ingredients to work their magic. It's essential to relax and breathe deeply during the bath to enhance the calming effects. After soaking, rinse off with clean water and pat dry with a towel.

Side Effects: Detox baths are generally safe for most people when used as directed, but some individuals may experience skin irritation or allergic reactions to certain ingredients. It's essential to perform a patch test before using new ingredients and discontinue use if any adverse reactions occur. Additionally, pregnant or breastfeeding women, individuals with certain medical conditions, or those taking medications should consult with a healthcare provider before using detox baths.

Detox Teas:

Definition: Detox teas are herbal teas or blends formulated with ingredients believed to support the body's detoxification processes, aid digestion, promote weight loss, and boost overall health.

Ingredients: Detox teas may contain a variety of ingredients such as green tea, dandelion, milk thistle, ginger, licorice root, peppermint, cinnamon, and various herbs and botanicals known for their detoxifying and digestive properties.

How to Prepare: Preparing detox tea involves steeping the tea bag or loose tea leaves in hot water for several minutes, typically 5 to 10 minutes, to allow the flavors and beneficial compounds to infuse into the water. Some detox teas may be consumed hot or cold, depending on personal preference.

Dosage: The recommended dosage of detox tea can vary depending on the specific blend and individual tolerance. It's generally advisable to start with a single cup per day and gradually increase as desired, following the instructions provided on the tea packaging.

How to Use: Detox teas can be enjoyed at any time of day, but many people prefer to drink them in the morning or before meals to support digestion and metabolism. It's essential to listen to your body's cues and adjust the frequency of consumption based on how you feel.

Side Effects: While detox teas are generally considered safe for most people when consumed in moderation, some individuals may experience side effects such as gastrointestinal upset, including bloating, gas, or diarrhea, especially if sensitive to certain ingredients. Detox teas containing caffeine may also cause jitteriness or disrupt sleep in some individuals. It's important to read the ingredient list carefully and avoid detox teas containing ingredients that may interact with medications or exacerbate underlying health conditions. Pregnant or breastfeeding women, individuals with certain medical conditions, or those taking medications should consult with a healthcare provider before using detox teas.

Dry Skin Brushing:

Definition: Dry skin brushing is a self-care technique that involves using a natural bristle brush to gently massage the skin in a specific pattern to promote exfoliation, stimulate circulation, and support lymphatic drainage.

Ingredients: Dry skin brushing requires a natural bristle brush with a long handle for reaching all areas of the body.

How to Prepare: Preparing for dry skin brushing involves selecting a suitable brush with natural bristles and ensuring that the skin is dry and free from moisturizers or oils.

Dosage: There isn't a specific dosage for dry skin brushing, but it's generally recommended to brush the skin for a few minutes each day, preferably before bathing or showering, to reap the benefits.

How to Use: To use a dry skin brush, start at the feet and brush upwards towards the heart using gentle, circular motions. Continue brushing each area of the body, including the legs, arms, back, and abdomen, for several minutes. Avoid brushing over sensitive or broken skin areas.

Side Effects: Dry skin brushing is generally safe for most people when done correctly, but it may cause skin irritation or sensitivity in some individuals, especially those with sensitive skin or conditions such as eczema or psoriasis. It's essential to use gentle pressure and avoid brushing over areas of inflamed or broken skin. If irritation occurs, discontinue use and consult with a dermatologist.

Epsom Salt Baths:

Definition: Epsom salt baths involve adding Epsom salt, also known as magnesium sulfate, to a warm bath to help soothe sore muscles, relieve stress, promote relaxation, and potentially detoxify the body.

Ingredients: Epsom salt is the primary ingredient used in Epsom salt baths. It's a naturally occurring mineral compound composed of magnesium, sulfur, and oxygen.

How to Prepare: Preparing for an Epsom salt bath involves adding the desired amount of Epsom salt to a bathtub filled with warm water. The water temperature should be comfortable for soaking, and the Epsom salt should be thoroughly dissolved before entering the bath.

Dosage: The recommended dosage of Epsom salt for a bath can vary depending on individual preferences and needs. As a general guideline, adding 1 to 2 cups of Epsom salt to a standard-sized bathtub filled with warm water is typically sufficient for most people.

How to Use: To use an Epsom salt bath, simply immerse yourself in the tub and soak for 20 to 30 minutes or longer, allowing the Epsom salt to dissolve and infuse into the water. It's essential to relax and breathe deeply during the bath to maximize the calming effects. After soaking, rinse off with clean water and pat dry with a towel.

Side Effects: Epsom salt baths are generally safe for most people when used as directed, but some individuals may experience skin irritation or allergic reactions to Epsom salt. It's essential to perform a patch test before using Epsom salt baths and discontinue use if any adverse reactions occur. Pregnant or breastfeeding women, individuals with certain medical conditions, or those taking medications should consult with a healthcare provider before using Epsom salt baths. Additionally, it's important to stay hydrated during and after an Epsom salt bath to prevent dehydration.

Exercise:

Definition: Exercise refers to physical activity performed to improve health, fitness, or overall well-being. It encompasses a wide range of activities, including cardiovascular exercises, strength training, flexibility exercises, and balance exercises.

Ingredients: Exercise requires varying combinations of movements, depending on the specific type of activity. Examples include running, walking, cycling, swimming, weightlifting, yoga, Pilates, and dancing.

How to Prepare: Preparing for exercise involves selecting appropriate clothing and footwear, warming up with dynamic stretches or light cardio, and ensuring hydration and nutrition levels are adequate.

Dosage: The recommended dosage of exercise depends on factors such as age, fitness level, health status, and exercise goals. As a general guideline, adults should aim for at least 150 minutes of moderate-intensity aerobic activity or 75 minutes of vigorous-intensity aerobic activity per week, along with muscle-strengthening activities on two or more days per week.

How to Use: Exercise can be integrated into daily routines in various ways, such as walking or cycling for transportation, taking the stairs instead of the elevator, or participating in structured exercise sessions at a gym or fitness facility. It's important to choose activities that are enjoyable and sustainable to maintain long-term adherence.

Side Effects: While exercise offers numerous health benefits, including improved cardiovascular health, weight management, mood enhancement, and stress reduction, overexertion or improper technique can lead to injuries such as strains, sprains, or fractures. It's essential to listen to your body, start gradually, and seek guidance from qualified fitness professionals to minimize the risk of injury.

Fasting:

Definition: Fasting involves voluntarily abstaining from food and/or drink for a specified period, often for religious, spiritual, health, or weight loss purposes.

Ingredients: Fasting requires no specific ingredients, as it involves restricting food intake for a predetermined period.

How to Prepare: Preparing for a fast involves planning the duration and type of fast, ensuring adequate hydration, and considering any potential medical implications or contraindications.

Dosage: The duration and frequency of fasting can vary widely, ranging from intermittent fasting protocols lasting several hours to extended fasts lasting multiple days or weeks. It's essential to choose a fasting regimen that aligns with individual health goals and preferences and to consult with a healthcare professional if there are any concerns.

How to Use: Fasting protocols may involve various approaches, including intermittent fasting (e.g., 16/8 method, alternate-day fasting), time-restricted feeding, water fasting, juice fasting, or religious fasting practices. It's important to stay hydrated during fasting periods and to break the fast gradually to avoid digestive discomfort.

Side Effects: While fasting may offer potential health benefits such as improved metabolic health, weight loss, and cellular repair processes, it can also pose risks, especially for certain populations such as pregnant or breastfeeding women, individuals with medical conditions such as diabetes or eating disorders, and those taking medications. Side effects of fasting may include dehydration, low blood sugar, headaches, dizziness, fatigue, irritability, and difficulty concentrating. It's essential to approach fasting mindfully, listen to your body's cues, and seek guidance from a healthcare professional before embarking on any fasting regimen, particularly if you have underlying health concerns.

Foot Detox Pads:

Definition: Foot detox pads are adhesive patches that are applied to the soles of the feet overnight. They are believed to help draw out toxins from the body through the feet while you sleep, promoting detoxification and overall wellness.

Ingredients: Foot detox pads typically contain a combination of natural ingredients such as bamboo vinegar, tourmaline, herbs (e.g., ginger, lavender, mint), and other botanical extracts. These ingredients are believed to have detoxifying properties and help absorb toxins from the body.

How to Prepare: Preparing for foot detox pad application involves cleansing and drying the feet thoroughly before bedtime. The pads are then applied to the soles of the feet, preferably on the reflexology points, and left on overnight.

Dosage: The frequency of foot detox pad use can vary depending on individual preferences and needs. Some people may use them nightly, while others may use them a few times a week or less frequently.

How to Use: To use foot detox pads, simply adhere them to the clean, dry soles of your feet before bedtime. Wear socks over the pads to keep them in place overnight. In the morning, remove the pads and discard them. Some pads may change color or appear darker after use, which is often attributed to the absorption of toxins from the body.

Side Effects: While foot detox pads are generally considered safe for most people, some individuals may experience skin irritation or allergic reactions to certain ingredients in the pads. It's essential to perform a patch test before using foot detox pads extensively and discontinue use if any adverse reactions occur. Additionally, foot detox pads may not be suitable for individuals with sensitive skin or certain medical conditions, so it's advisable to consult with a healthcare provider before using them, especially if you have concerns.

Kale Mango Smoothie

Definition: A kale mango smoothie is a blended beverage that combines the nutrient-rich kale with the tropical sweetness of mango. This smoothie is known for its vibrant color and refreshing taste, offering a wealth of vitamins, minerals, and antioxidants.

Ingredients: Typical ingredients for a kale mango smoothie include fresh kale leaves (stems removed), ripe mango chunks, a liquid base such as coconut water or almond milk, a source of creaminess like Greek yogurt or avocado, and optional additions like honey or lime juice for added flavor.

How to Prepare: To prepare a kale mango smoothie, simply combine the kale leaves, mango chunks, liquid base, source of creaminess, and any optional additions in a blender. Blend until smooth and creamy, adjusting the quantities of each ingredient to achieve your desired taste and consistency.

Dosage: There is no strict dosage for consuming kale mango smoothies, but incorporating them into your daily diet as a nutritious snack or meal replacement can be beneficial. Enjoy one serving per day or as desired.

How to Use: Enjoy a kale mango smoothie as a refreshing breakfast option, a post-workout snack, or a light and hydrating dessert. It can also be incorporated into a detox or cleansing regimen for added health benefits.

Side Effects: Kale mango smoothies are generally safe for most people when consumed in moderation. However, some individuals may experience digestive discomfort if kale is consumed in large quantities or if they have a sensitivity to certain compounds in mango. Additionally, individuals taking blood thinners should be cautious with kale consumption due to its vitamin K content.

Lemon Lime Cucumber Smoothie

Definition: A lemon lime cucumber smoothie is a blended beverage that combines the citrusy flavors of lemon and lime with the refreshing crispness of cucumber. This smoothie is known for its hydrating properties and bright, tangy taste.

Ingredients: Common ingredients for a lemon lime cucumber smoothie include peeled and sliced cucumber, freshly squeezed lemon and lime juice, a liquid base such as water or coconut water, a source of sweetness like honey or agave syrup, and optional additions like mint leaves or ginger for added flavor.

How to Prepare: To prepare a lemon lime cucumber smoothie, simply combine the sliced cucumber, lemon and lime juice, liquid base, source of sweetness, and any optional additions in a blender. Blend until smooth and creamy, adjusting the quantities of each ingredient to achieve your desired taste and consistency.

Dosage: There is no strict dosage for consuming lemon lime cucumber smoothies, but incorporating them into your daily diet as a hydrating beverage or refreshing snack can be beneficial. Enjoy one serving per day or as desired.

How to Use: Enjoy a lemon lime cucumber smoothie as a revitalizing breakfast option, a post-workout snack, or a light and refreshing drink on a hot day. It can also be incorporated into a detox or cleansing regimen for added health benefits.

Side Effects: Lemon lime cucumber smoothies are generally safe for most people when consumed in moderation. However, individuals with citrus allergies or sensitivities may experience adverse reactions. Additionally, some people may experience digestive discomfort if cucumber is consumed in large quantities.

Lettuce Orange Smoothie

Definition: A lettuce orange smoothie is a blended beverage that combines the crisp freshness of lettuce with the citrusy sweetness of oranges. This smoothie offers a unique flavor profile and a wealth of vitamins, minerals, and antioxidants, making it a refreshing and nutritious option for any time of day.

Ingredients: Typical ingredients for a lettuce orange smoothie include fresh lettuce leaves (such as romaine or green leaf lettuce), peeled and segmented oranges, a liquid base such as orange juice or coconut water, a source of creaminess like Greek yogurt or banana, and optional additions like honey or ginger for added flavor.

How to Prepare: To prepare a lettuce orange smoothie, simply combine the lettuce leaves, orange segments, liquid base, source of creaminess, and any optional additions in a blender. Blend until smooth and creamy, adjusting the quantities of each ingredient to achieve your desired taste and consistency.

Dosage: There is no strict dosage for consuming lettuce orange smoothies, but incorporating them into your daily diet as a nutritious snack or meal replacement can be beneficial. Enjoy one serving per day or as desired.

How to Use: Enjoy a lettuce orange smoothie as a refreshing breakfast option, a post-workout snack, or a light and hydrating dessert. It can also be incorporated into a detox or cleansing regimen for added health benefits.

Side Effects: Lettuce orange smoothies are generally safe for most people when consumed in moderation. However, some individuals may be allergic to certain types of lettuce or experience digestive discomfort if lettuce is consumed in large quantities. Additionally, individuals with citrus allergies should be cautious with orange consumption.

Moringa Pineapple Smoothie

Definition: A moringa pineapple smoothie is a blended beverage that combines the nutrient-rich moringa powder with the tropical sweetness of pineapple. This smoothie is packed with vitamins, minerals, and antioxidants, making it a nutritious and energizing option for promoting overall health and well-being.

Ingredients: Common ingredients for a moringa pineapple smoothie include moringa powder, fresh or frozen pineapple chunks, a liquid base such as coconut water or almond milk, a source of creaminess like Greek yogurt or avocado, and optional additions like spinach or mango for added nutrition and flavor.

How to Prepare: To prepare a moringa pineapple smoothie, simply combine the moringa powder, pineapple chunks, liquid base, source of creaminess, and any optional additions in a blender. Blend until smooth and creamy, adjusting the quantities of each ingredient to achieve your desired taste and consistency.

Dosage: There is no strict dosage for consuming moringa pineapple smoothies, but incorporating them into your daily diet as a nutritious snack or meal replacement can be beneficial. Enjoy one serving per day or as desired.

How to Use: Enjoy a moringa pineapple smoothie as a revitalizing breakfast option, a post-workout snack, or a nutrient-packed meal replacement. It can also be incorporated into a detox or cleansing regimen for added health benefits.

Side Effects: Moringa pineapple smoothies are generally safe for most people when consumed in moderation. However, some individuals may be sensitive to moringa or experience digestive discomfort if pineapple is consumed in large quantities. Additionally, individuals taking certain medications or with certain medical conditions should consult with a healthcare professional before consuming moringa regularly.

Nopal Pear Smoothie

Definition: A nopal pear smoothie is a blended beverage that combines the unique flavor and texture of nopales (prickly pear cactus pads) with the sweetness of pears. This smoothie offers a refreshing taste and a range of potential health benefits, including hydration, fiber, and essential nutrients.

Ingredients: Typical ingredients for a nopal pear smoothie include chopped nopales (prickly pear cactus pads), ripe pear slices, a liquid base such as water or coconut water, a source of creaminess like Greek yogurt or avocado, and optional additions like lime juice or honey for added flavor.

How to Prepare: To prepare a nopal pear smoothie, simply combine the chopped nopales, pear slices, liquid base, source of creaminess, and any optional additions in a blender. Blend until smooth and creamy, adjusting the quantities of each ingredient to achieve your desired taste and consistency.

Dosage: There is no strict dosage for consuming nopal pear smoothies, but incorporating them into your daily diet as a nutritious snack or meal replacement can be beneficial. Enjoy one serving per day or as desired.

How to Use: Enjoy a nopal pear smoothie as a refreshing breakfast option, a post-workout snack, or a light and hydrating dessert. It can also be incorporated into a detox or cleansing regimen for added health benefits.

Side Effects: Nopal pear smoothies are generally safe for most people when consumed in moderation. However, some individuals may be allergic to nopales or experience digestive discomfort if they have a sensitivity to certain compounds in pears. Additionally, individuals with certain medical conditions or taking certain medications should consult with a healthcare professional before consuming nopales regularly.

Okra Peach Smoothie

Definition: An okra peach smoothie is a blended beverage that combines the mild flavor of okra with the sweet juiciness of peaches. This smoothie offers a unique combination of flavors and textures along with a range of potential health benefits, including fiber, vitamins, and antioxidants.

Ingredients: Common ingredients for an okra peach smoothie include sliced okra pods, ripe peach slices, a liquid base such as almond milk or peach juice, a source of creaminess like Greek yogurt or banana, and optional additions like vanilla extract or cinnamon for added flavor.

How to Prepare: To prepare an okra peach smoothie, simply combine the sliced okra pods, peach slices, liquid base, source of creaminess, and any optional additions in a blender. Blend until smooth and creamy, adjusting the quantities of each ingredient to achieve your desired taste and consistency.

Dosage: There is no strict dosage for consuming okra peach smoothies, but incorporating them into your daily diet as a nutritious snack or meal replacement can be beneficial. Enjoy one serving per day or as desired.

How to Use: Enjoy an okra peach smoothie as a satisfying breakfast option, a post-workout snack, or a nutrient-packed meal replacement. It can also be incorporated into a detox or cleansing regimen for added health benefits.

Side Effects: Okra peach smoothies are generally safe for most people when consumed in moderation. However, some individuals may be sensitive to the mucilage (slimy substance) found in okra or experience digestive discomfort if they have a sensitivity to certain compounds in peaches. Additionally, individuals with certain medical conditions or taking certain medications should consult with a healthcare professional before consuming okra regularly.

Orange Turmeric Smoothie

Definition: An orange turmeric smoothie is a blended beverage that combines the citrusy sweetness of oranges with the earthy warmth of turmeric. This smoothie offers a burst of flavor along with potential health benefits from the anti-inflammatory properties of turmeric and the vitamin C content of oranges.

Ingredients: Typical ingredients for an orange turmeric smoothie include freshly squeezed orange juice, ground turmeric, a liquid base such as coconut water or almond milk, a source of creaminess like Greek yogurt or banana, and optional additions like black pepper or honey for enhanced absorption and flavor.

How to Prepare: To prepare an orange turmeric smoothie, simply combine the orange juice, ground turmeric, liquid base, source of creaminess, and any optional additions in a blender. Blend until smooth and creamy, adjusting the quantities of each ingredient to achieve your desired taste and consistency.

Dosage: There is no strict dosage for consuming orange turmeric smoothies, but incorporating them into your daily diet as a nutritious snack or meal replacement can be beneficial. Enjoy one serving per day or as desired.

How to Use: Enjoy an orange turmeric smoothie as a refreshing breakfast option, a post-workout snack, or a light and hydrating dessert. It can also be incorporated into a detox or cleansing regimen for added health benefits.

Side Effects: Orange turmeric smoothies are generally safe for most people when consumed in moderation. However, some individuals may experience digestive discomfort if they are sensitive to turmeric or have certain medical conditions. Additionally, turmeric may interact with certain medications, so individuals taking medications should consult with a healthcare professional before consuming turmeric regularly.

Peach Ginger Smoothie

Definition: A peach ginger smoothie is a blended beverage that combines the sweet flavor of peaches with the spicy warmth of ginger. This smoothie offers a delightful balance of flavors along with potential health benefits from the anti-inflammatory properties of ginger and the vitamins and minerals found in peaches.

Ingredients: Common ingredients for a peach ginger smoothie include ripe peach slices, peeled and grated ginger root, a liquid base such as coconut water or orange juice, a source of creaminess like Greek yogurt or banana, and optional additions like honey or cinnamon for added flavor.

How to Prepare: To prepare a peach ginger smoothie, simply combine the peach slices, grated ginger, liquid base, source of creaminess, and any optional additions in a blender. Blend until smooth and creamy, adjusting the quantities of each ingredient to achieve your desired taste and consistency.

Dosage: There is no strict dosage for consuming peach ginger smoothies, but incorporating them into your daily diet as a nutritious snack or meal replacement can be beneficial. Enjoy one serving per day or as desired.

How to Use: Enjoy a peach ginger smoothie as a refreshing breakfast option, a post-workout snack, or a light and energizing dessert. It can also be incorporated into a detox or cleansing regimen for added health benefits.

Side Effects: Peach ginger smoothies are generally safe for most people when consumed in moderation. However, some individuals may be sensitive to ginger or experience digestive discomfort if ginger is consumed in large quantities. Additionally, some people may be allergic to peaches, so be cautious if you have any food allergies.

Ginger Tea:

Definition: Ginger tea is a hot beverage made from fresh or dried ginger root steeped in hot water. It's known for its spicy, aromatic flavor and potential health benefits.

Ingredients: Ginger tea is made primarily from ginger root and water. Some people may also add other ingredients such as lemon, honey, or mint for flavor enhancement.

How to Prepare: Preparing ginger tea involves slicing, grating, or crushing fresh ginger root and steeping it in hot water for several minutes. Alternatively, dried ginger root or ginger tea bags can be used. The tea can be sweetened with honey or flavored with lemon, if desired.

Dosage: There isn't a specific dosage for ginger tea, but it's generally safe to consume in moderation. One to three cups of ginger tea per day is often recommended to reap its potential health benefits.

How to Use: Ginger tea can be enjoyed hot or cold, depending on personal preference. It can be consumed on its own or combined with other ingredients such as lemon or honey for added flavor. Some people enjoy ginger tea as a soothing beverage in the morning or as a digestive aid after meals.

Side Effects: Ginger tea is generally well-tolerated by most people when consumed in moderation, but some individuals may experience side effects such as heartburn, stomach upset, or diarrhea, especially when consumed in large quantities. It may also interact with certain medications, such as blood thinners or diabetes medications, so it's advisable to consult with a healthcare provider before consuming ginger tea regularly, especially if you have underlying health conditions or are taking medications.

Green Smoothies:

Definition: Green smoothies are blended beverages made primarily from leafy green vegetables, fruits, and other nutritious ingredients. They are popular for their health benefits and versatility.

Ingredients: Green smoothies typically include leafy greens such as spinach, kale, or Swiss chard, along with fruits like bananas, apples, berries, or mangoes. Other common ingredients may include vegetables (e.g., cucumber, celery), herbs (e.g., parsley, cilantro), liquids (e.g., water, coconut water, almond milk), and optional add-ins such as protein powder, chia seeds, or nut butter.

How to Prepare: Preparing a green smoothie involves combining the desired ingredients in a blender and blending until smooth and creamy. The ratio of greens to fruits and other ingredients can be adjusted according to personal taste preferences and nutritional goals.

Dosage: There isn't a specific dosage for green smoothies, but incorporating them into your diet regularly can provide numerous health benefits. Aim to consume one or more servings of green smoothies per day as part of a balanced diet.

How to Use: Green smoothies can be enjoyed as a nutritious breakfast, snack, or post-workout refresher. They are convenient and portable, making them an excellent option for busy lifestyles. Experiment with different combinations of ingredients to create your favorite flavor combinations.

Side Effects: Green smoothies are generally considered safe for most people when made with fresh, whole ingredients. However, some individuals may experience digestive upset or bloating, especially if they're not accustomed to consuming large amounts of fiber-rich foods. It's essential to start with small portions and gradually increase the amount of greens in your smoothies to allow your body to adjust. If you have specific health concerns or dietary restrictions, consult with a healthcare provider or registered dietitian before making significant changes to your diet.

Body Brushing:

Definition: Body brushing, also known as dry brushing, is a self-care practice that involves using a natural bristle brush to exfoliate the skin and stimulate circulation.

Ingredients: Body brushing requires only a natural bristle brush with a long handle for reaching the back and other areas of the body.

How to Prepare: Preparing for body brushing involves selecting a suitable brush with natural bristles and ensuring the skin is dry and free from moisturizers or oils.

Dosage: There isn't a specific dosage for body brushing, but it's typically done once a day or a few times a week as part of a skincare routine.

How to Use: To use a body brush, start at the feet and brush upwards towards the heart using gentle, circular motions. Continue brushing each area of the body, including the legs, arms, back, and abdomen, for several minutes. Avoid brushing over sensitive or broken skin areas.

Side Effects: Body brushing is generally safe for most people when done correctly, but it may cause skin irritation or sensitivity in some individuals, especially those with sensitive skin or conditions such as eczema or psoriasis. It's essential to use gentle pressure and avoid brushing over areas of inflamed or broken skin. If irritation occurs, discontinue use and consult with a dermatologist. Additionally, body brushing may not be suitable for individuals with certain medical conditions such as varicose veins or open wounds, so it's advisable to consult with a healthcare provider before starting this practice.

THE END